Eat your
Super hero foods
Alexis!

G

SUPER HERO FOODS
★ and the ABCs of Nutrition ★

by Greg Crawford
HealthyKidsofAmerica.org

FEATURING...

★ **C**ALCIUM ★

★ *I*ODINE ★

★ **I**RON ★

★ **O**MEGA 3 (GOOD FAT) ★

★ **M**AGNESIUM ★

★ **P**OTASSIUM ★

★ VITAMIN **A** (BETA-CAROTENE) ★

★ **B** VITAMINS ★

★ **VITAMIN** *C* ★

★ VITAMIN **D** ★

★ **VITAMIN** **E** ★

★ VITAMIN **K** ★

★ **Z**INC ★

AND THE

SUPER HERO

Foods!

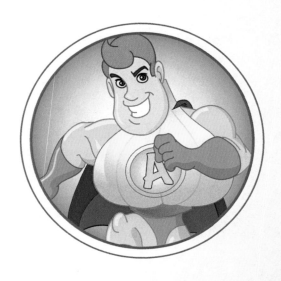

Healthy Kids of America
(a non-profit organization)

www.thesuperherofoods.com
www.healthykidsofamerica.org
phone: 973-267-2121

OUR MISSION: To plant a seed in the mind of young kids about the importance of good nutrition and fitness, with the purpose of taking control of our country's health epidemic.

It is our belief that by educating our kids about the importance of nutrition and fitness at a young age, they will make better choices for their health in the future.

OUR ORGANIZATION PROVIDES:

- A team of nutritionists that provide on-site and easy to understand nutrition course for kids

- On site education for parents on what and how to feed their children, and how to cook *healthy yet tasty*

- Fitness classes for kids that focus on basic movement functions and safe exercises designed to increase the child's awareness of different fitness modalities

- On site healthy vending machine and food options for local schools in the community

- A charity that benefits YOU and YOUR kids

TABLE OF CONTENTS

Who wants to have more energy, grow to be strong, improve memory, be able to focus, and just be **SUPER HEALTHY?**

The mission of this book is to plant a seed in the mind of young kids about the importance of good nutrition, with the purpose of taking control of our country's health epidemic. It is our belief that by educating our kids about the importance of nutrition at a young age, they will make better choices for their health in the future.

The way you look at food and what it contains is going to shape the way you grow up and become a healthy adult. There has to be a balance when it comes to food—part enjoyment, part feeding hunger, and part nourishment and fuel.

The nourishment and fuel is the most important aspect, and if you understand this importance, then you will grow up to be a smarter, stronger, healthier and happier person.

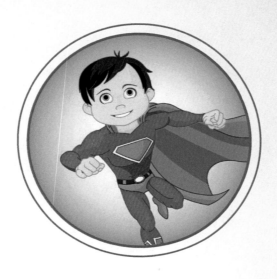

This book is broken down into five sections:

This book starts with two simple lessons about nutrition. In Chapter 3, you'll meet **The Super Hero Foods.** These illustrated characters (and their rivals, *the Villains*) present a fun way for kids to remember and expand their knowledge of nutrition. There are quizzes and challenges through out this book to see how much of the information you've absorbed. At the end of this book, you'll find recipes and resources to inspire you to make a positive change in your family's diet.

Small changes can make a **Super** difference!

WATER

- 60% of our bodies are water.
- Water is involved with almost every function of the body.
- Water carries all the ABC's of nutrition throughout our body.

VITAMINS & MINERALS

VITAMINS

Vitamins are essential for growth, vitality and health, and are helpful in digestion, elimination, and resistance to disease. Depletions or deficiencies can lead to a variety of both specific nutritional disorders and general health problems, depending on what vitamin is lacking in the diet.

Water-soluble vitamins

Includes the B vitamins and vitamin *C*. They are mainly found in raw vegetable foods but can be lost easily during cooking or processing.

Water-soluble vitamins are not stored in the body, so they are needed regularly. They are generally not toxic when taken in excess.

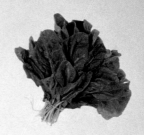

B VITAMINS

- There are 14 total **B** vitamins.
- The **B** vitamins are all related and work together, so it is suggested to keep them in balance which we call the "The B Complex."

Where it is found

Found mainly in the germ of grains, some beans and nuts and leafy vegetables.

Benefits

- Known as the spark plugs of the body, they support many functions.
- Helps provide energy and relaxation.
- Helps your body use carbohydrates, proteins, and fats properly.

VITAMIN *C*

- C stands for citrus, where the vitamin is mostly found.
- Known as "The Healthy Vitamin"

Where it is found

You find vitamin *C* only in raw fruits and vegetables.

Benefits

- Works in the formation of collagen. Collagen is needed to keep skin strong, heal wounds and maintain healthy blood vessels.
- Helps some of the **B** vitamins form important brain chemicals and hormones.
- Helps in lowering cholesterol.
- Reduces toxins in the body.
- Boosts your immune system.

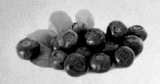
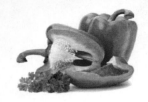

Fat-soluble vitamins

Includes vitamins **A**, **D**, **E**, and **K**. They are found in both vegetables and animals.

They can be stored in the body, so they can function for a longer time. Toxic levels can occur if taken in excess, especially vitamin **A**, **D** and **K**.

VITAMIN A (BETA-CAROTENE)

- Fat-soluble
- Comes in the form of beta-carotene or Retinol

Where it is found

Vitamin **A** is mostly found in liver, sweet potato, carrots, dark leafy greens, butternut squash, lettuce, cantaloupe, dried apricots, paprika, red pepper, cayenne, and chili powder.

Benefits

- Helps protect eyesight
- Promotes growth and tissue healing
- Healthy skin
- Lowers risk of cancer

VITAMIN D

- Fat-soluble
- Known as "sunshine" vitamin because it can be made in the skin from the sun's rays

Where it is found

Vitamin **D** is found in milk, eggs, sardines, and also in sun exposure.

Benefits

- Helps regulate calcium for strong bones and healthy teeth
- Promotes growth

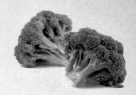

VITAMIN E

- Fat-soluble
- An antioxidant vitamin

Where it is found

Nuts are one of the best sources of vitamin E, including almonds and peanuts, sunflower seeds, green leafy vegetables, and vegetable oils.

Benefits

- Helps prevent cancer
- Healthy skin
- Protects the arteries and heart

VITAMIN K

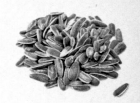

- Fat-soluble
- The blood clotting vitamin

Where it is found

Vitamin K is found mostly in leafy green vegetables, cauliflower, tomatoes, and blueberries.

Benefits

- Needed to stop bleeding

MINERALS

Minerals are just as important as vitamins and some-times harder to get since there are only trace amounts found in the foods we eat. We are all made up of minerals which are elements that come from the earth. These elements make up our bodies. Minerals are essential to our physical and mental health.

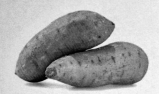

There are approximately 17 essential minerals. Many of the minerals work together with different vitamins to perform a function.

In this book you will learn about six of the most popular, common minerals.

CALCIUM

- Most abundant and one of the most important
- Calcium works with other vitamins and minerals like vitamin D, Phosphorus, and Magnesium. Needs vitamin D to be used in the body.
- Vitamin D is its power booster

Powers

- Best known for the development and strength of bones and teeth – works with vitamin D and Phosphorus
- Calcium is needed for muscles to flex and the heart to beat – with Magnesium
- Needed for your nerves to signal
- Lowers risk of cancer

MAGNESIUM

- Known as the calming mineral

Powers

- Helps relax the muscles
- Important for energy production
- Calms the nerves

POTASSIUM

- Known as an electrolyte
- Works opposite of Sodium.

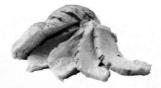

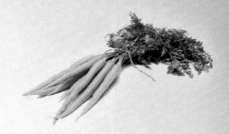

Powers

- Balances water in the body with Sodium. Most of our diets are too high in Sodium and too low in Potassium.
- Helps with electric charge for nerves in the body
- Aids in the use of proteins and carbohydrates

Sodium

- Found highly in the Villain food group – *Salty*
- Works against Potassium.
- Too much is bad for the fluids in the body, causing high blood pressure.

IRON

- The main use of Iron is to help carry oxygen in the blood to important parts of the body.
- Some people are low in Iron which is called Anemia. It is very common especially in women and people with poor diets.
- Low Iron leads to low energy – making you tired.

ZINC

- Best known as the most underrated mineral
- Zinc is found in the body in small amounts but has many functions.

Powers

- Immune system support
- Enhances wound or burn feeling
- It is good for skin and hair
- Helps aid in growth and reproduction (having babies)

QUIZ:
Chapter 1

NAME ————————————

DATE ————————————

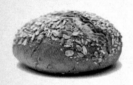

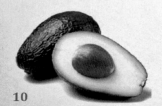

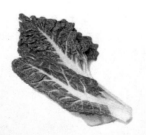

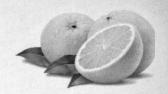

What did you learn?

1. Our bodies are made up mostly of _____.

2. Name the 2 different categories of vitamins.

_____   _____

3. There were 6 minerals discussed. Name 3.

_____   _____   _____

4. Where can you find vitamin C?

_____

5. Which vitamin gives you energy?

_____

6. What is Calcium best known for?

_____

7. What is your favorite fruit? _____
Which do you want to try? _____

8. What is your favorite vegetable? _____
Which do you want to try? _____

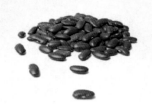

THE FOOD NUTRIENTS (Protein, Carbohydrates, and Fat)

PROTEIN

The most important nutrient group, this type of food should be on your plate at every main meal.

Protein is needed for the growth and maintenance of the body tissues and is very important during childhood. It is primarily important for growth of:

- Muscles
- Hair
- Nails
- Skin
- Organs

Protein is also required by our immune system to protect us from infections. Protein mostly consists of:

- Dairy – eggs, yogurt, cheese, milk
- Meat – chicken, lean beef, turkey
- Fish – tilapia, halibut, flounder, salmon, tuna, whiting, bass, snapper
- Beans/Legumes – kidney, black, lima, pinto, red, lentils, chickpeas
- Nuts – almonds, walnuts, pecans, edamame

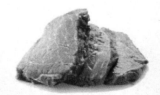

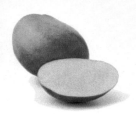
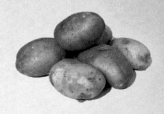

CARBOHYDRATES

Carbohydrates are a source of energy for the body. They break down into sugar in the body known as "glucose".

Carbohydrates come in 3 forms:

- Simple sugar (table sugar, candy, milk, cereals, white bread) – can be really bad for your body
- Fructose (fruit)
- Starches/grains (rice, potato, pasta) – *Multi grain/whole wheat is best*

Carbohydrates are stored in the muscles, liver or as body fat. Too much high sugar carbohydrates could lead to more being stored as body fat.

Fiber – found in some carbohydrates like fruits and some starches/grains – slows down the sugar being stored as body fat.

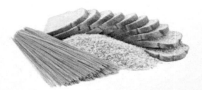

FATS

DON'T BE AFRAID OF FAT. (Just know what's good and what's bad).

Bad fats – saturated and trans (think butter and lard) raise the levels of bad cholesterol and contain more cholesterol.

Examples:

– Processed foods:
- Cakes
- Muffins
- Donuts
- Cookies
- Pies
- Chips
- Butter
- Salad dressing
- Mayonnaise

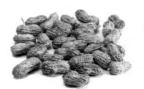

– Dairy and fatty meat

– Deep fried vegetable oils contain saturated fats

Good fats – Unsaturated

Examples:

- Some oils such as:
- Olive
- Canola
- Peanut
- Sunflower
- Sesame
- Soybean
- Corn
- Safflower

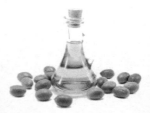

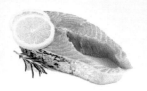

– Fatty fish: (very high in OMEGA 3 and 6 Fatty acids which is what we NEED)

- Salmon
- Mackerel
- Herring
- Trout

– Nuts: (unsalted)

- Almonds
- Walnuts
- Pecans
- Cashews

– Peanut butter

– Avocado

– Seeds: (unsalted)

- Pumpkin
- Sunflower

– Coconut (unsweetened)

Your body uses the **good (unsaturated) fats** to help with:

- Hormone production
- Energy source
- Anti-inflammatory
- Blood thinner
- Nerve function

We need some of the good and none of the bad!

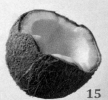

QUIZ:
Chapter 2

NAME _____

DATE _____

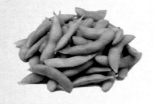

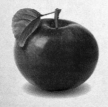

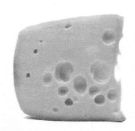

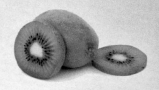

What did you learn?

1. Name the 3 types of food discussed in Chapter 2:

P_____   C_____   F_____

2. What are the two types of fats?

_____   _____

3. Give an example of a *simple sugar:*

_____

4. Name 3 examples of *good fats:*

_____   _____   _____

5. Which type of food should you have with every meal?

_____

CHALLENGE:

Name one healthy *protein* source that you would enjoy with each meal of the day:

Breakfast: _____

Lunch: _____

Dinner: _____

AND NOW... THE
SUPER HERO
Foods!

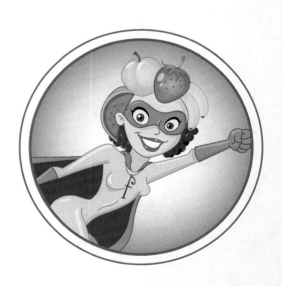

THE GREEN CRUCIFEROUS MAN

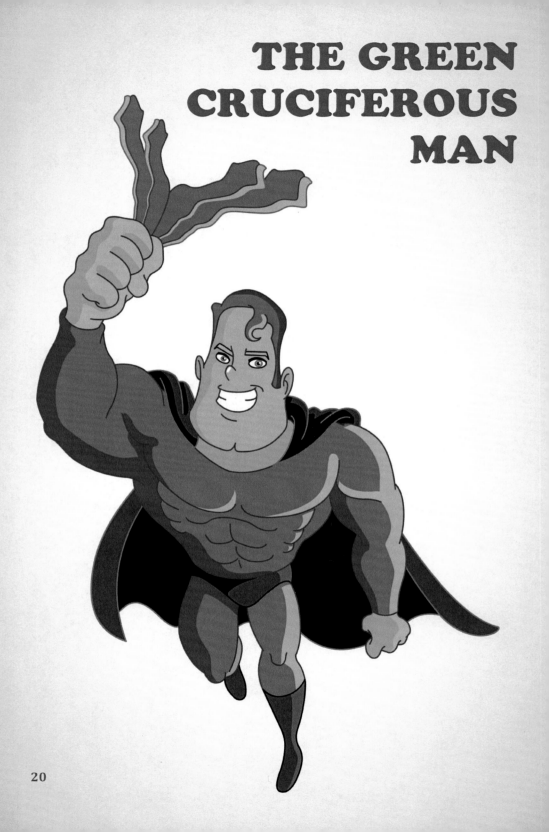

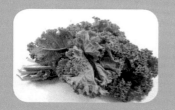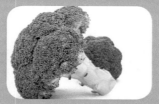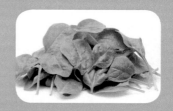

SUPER HERO FOOD 1:

The Green Cruciferous Man

Where to find him...
★ Kale
★ Broccoli
★ Cabbage
★ Spinach
★ Lettuce
★ Cauliflower

His Weapons...
★ Vitamin C
★ Vitamin A
★ Vitamin E
★ Magnesium
★ Calcium
★ Iron

His Powers... (the MOST POWERFUL of the Super Hero foods!)
★ Fights cancer
★ Anti-aging powers
★ Strengthens bones
★ Stronger muscles
★ Prevents disease (heart disease, diabetes, arthritis)

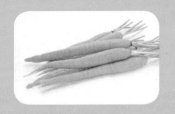 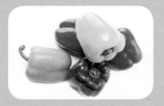 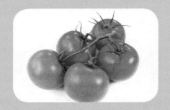

Carotenoid Man

Where to find him...
★ Carrots
★ Bell peppers
★ Sweet potatoes
★ Squash
★ Tomatoes

His Weapons...
★ Vitamin C
★ B Vitamins
★ Vitamin A (Beta-Carotene)
★ Potassium

His Powers...
★ Fights off germs
★ Prevents disease (heart disease, diabetes, arthritis)
★ Protects vision

CAROTENOID MAN

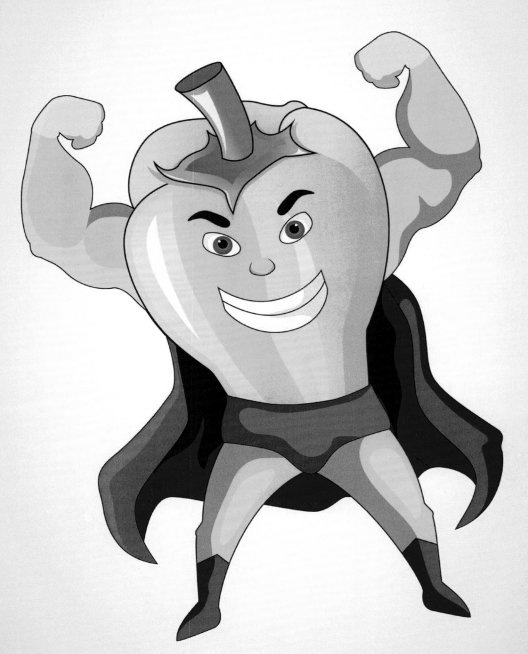

FRUITISHA

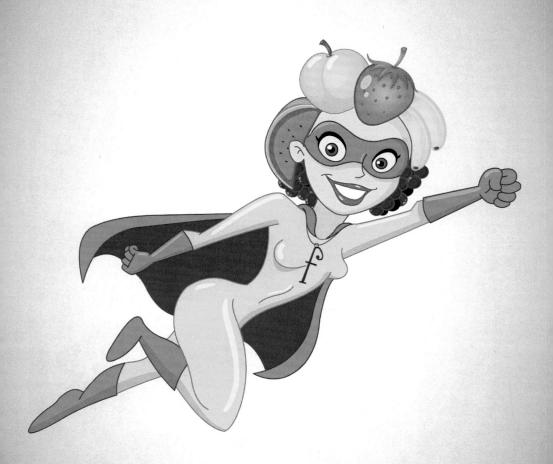

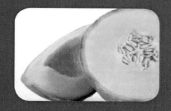 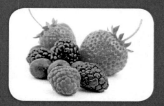 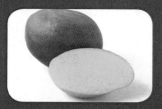

SUPER HERO FOOD 3:

Fruitisha

Where to find her...
★ Melons
★ Berries
★ Pineapple
★ Mango
★ Apples
★ Oranges

Her Weapons...
★ Vitamin C
★ Vitamin A
★ Vitamin E
★ B Vitamins
★ Calcium
★ Magnesium

Her Powers...
★ Fights germs
★ Super vision
★ Prevents diseases
★ Energizes

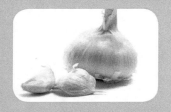 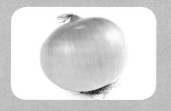 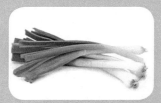

SUPER HERO FOOD 4:

Allium Al

Where to find him...
★ Onions
★ Garlic
★ Scallions

His Weapons...
★ Calcium
★ Potassium
★ Vitamin C
★ B Vitamins

His Powers...
★ Destroys evil cholesterol
★ Helps the heart
★ Fights infections

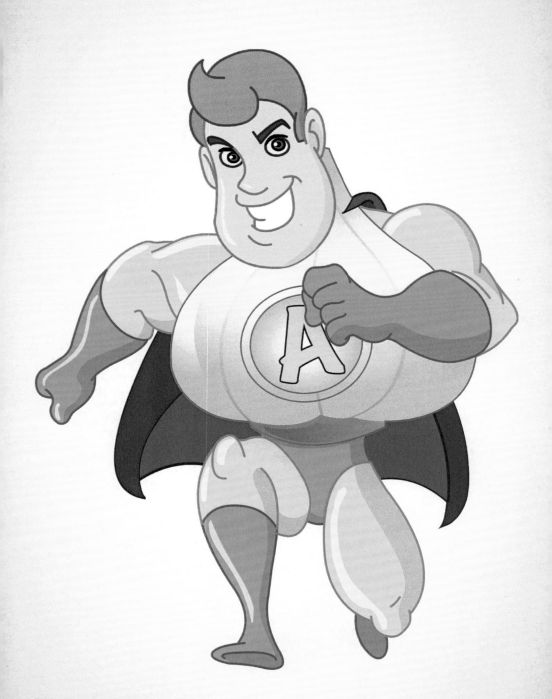

ALLIUM AL

SEAFOOD SULLY

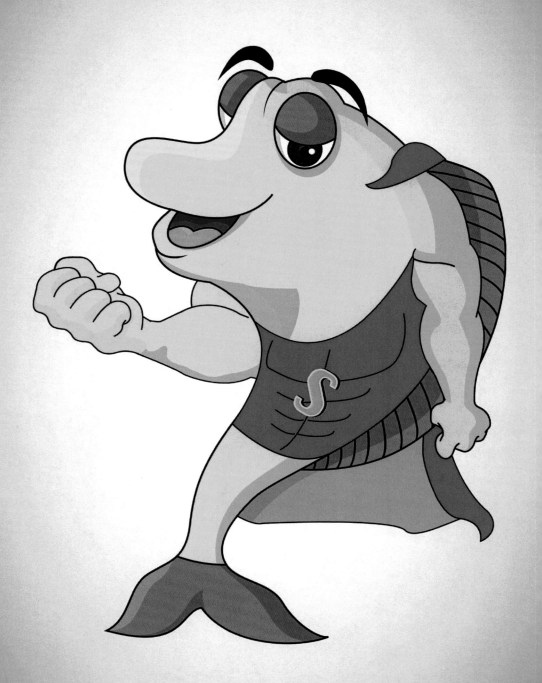

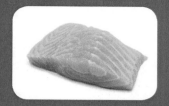 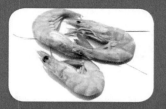 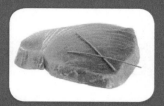

Seafood Sully

Where to find him...
★ Salmon
★ Tuna fish
★ Scallops
★ Lobster
★ Crab
★ Oysters
★ Shrimp

His Weapons...
★ Omega 3 (good fat)
★ Protein
★ Vitamin A
★ B Vitamins
★ Calcium
★ Iron
★ Magnesium
★ Potassium
★ Zinc
★ Iodine

His Powers...
★ Strengthens bones
★ Strong muscles
★ Gives energy
★ Destroys evil cholesterol

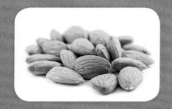 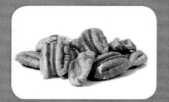 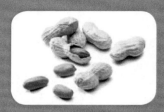

SUPER HERO FOOD 6:

Captain Nut

Where to find him...
★ Almonds
★ Walnuts
★ Pecans
★ Peanuts
★ Flax seed

His Weapons...
★ B Vitamins
★ Omega 3
★ Vitamin E
★ Calcium
★ Potassium

His Powers...
★ Gives energy
★ Strong heart
★ Destroys evil cholesterol

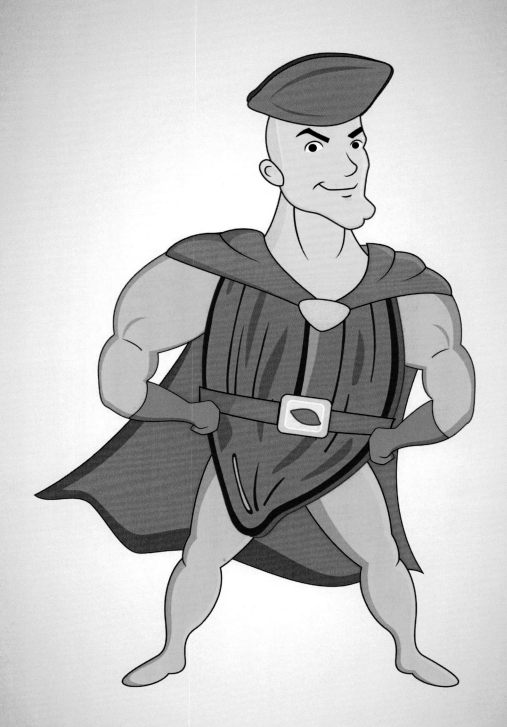

CAPTAIN NUT

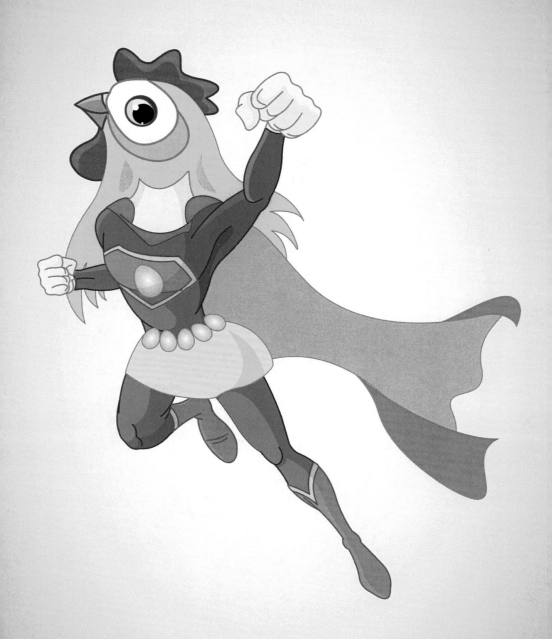

POULTRY PAM

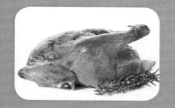 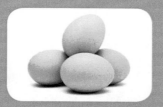 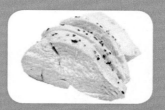

Poultry Pam

Where to find her...
★ Chickens (farm-raised and grass-fed, organic)
★ Eggs (organic)

Her Weapons...
★ Protein
★ Omega 3
★ Vitamin A
★ B Vitamins
★ Zinc

Her Powers...
★ Builds muscle and makes you strong
★ Gives energy

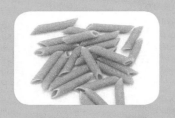 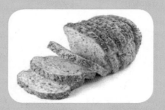 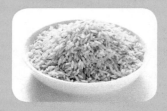

Whole Grain Harry

Where to find him...
★ Whole grain bread
★ Brown rice
★ Whole wheat pasta
★ Oatmeal

His Weapons...
★ B Vitamins
★ Vitamin E
★ Magnesium
★ Potassium
★ Zinc

His Powers...
★ He gives you long lasting energy
★ He makes you stronger
★ Be careful (too much of Whole Grain Harry is not good for you)

WHOLE GRAIN HARRY

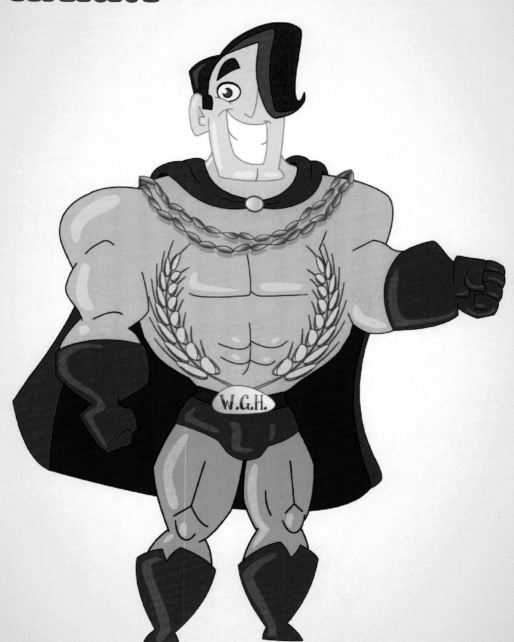

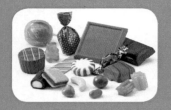 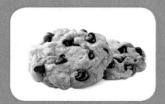 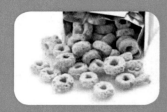

VILLAIN FOOD 1:

Shugar (sugar)

Where to find him...
✔ Candy
✔ White bread
✔ Ice cream
✔ Cookies
✔ Cereals
✔ Cake
✔ Soda
✔ Juice

His Powers...
✔ He will pretend to give you energy, then zap you of your energy
✔ He takes all your powers away from the Super Hero Foods
✔ Will put fat on your body
✔ Weakens your muscles

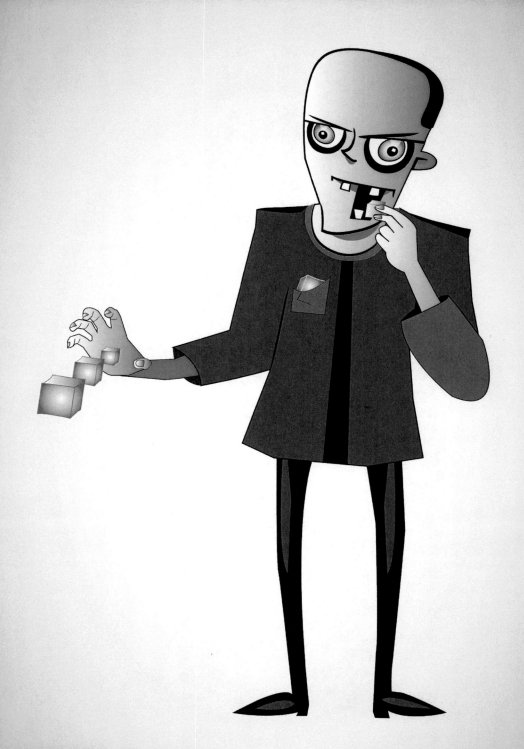

SHUGAR

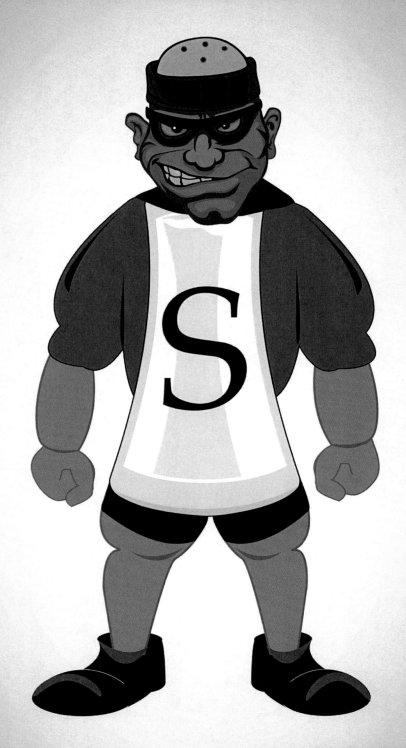

SALTY

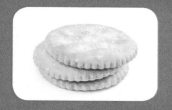 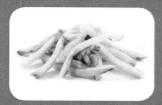 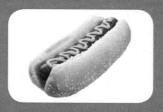

VILLAIN FOOD 2:

Salty

Where to find him...
✔ Pretzels
✔ Crackers
✔ Processed meats
✔ Soda
✔ Hot dogs
✔ French fries

His Powers...
✔ Takes water from your body
✔ Bad for your heart
✔ Fills you with evil cholesterol

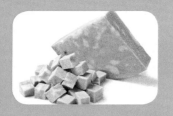
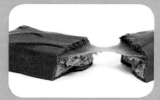
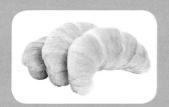

VILLAIN FOOD 3:

Processed Pete

Where to find him...
✔ Cold-cut meats
✔ Canned foods
✔ Breads
✔ Candy bars
✔ Cereals

His Powers...
✔ He contains chemicals your body cannot digest
✔ He takes all your powers away from the Super Hero Foods
✔ He will pretend to give you energy, then zap you of your energy
✔ He will cause disease

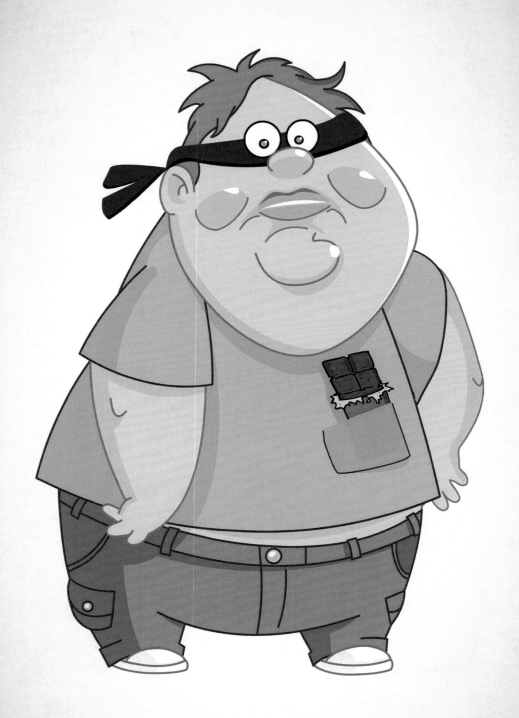

PROCESSED PETE

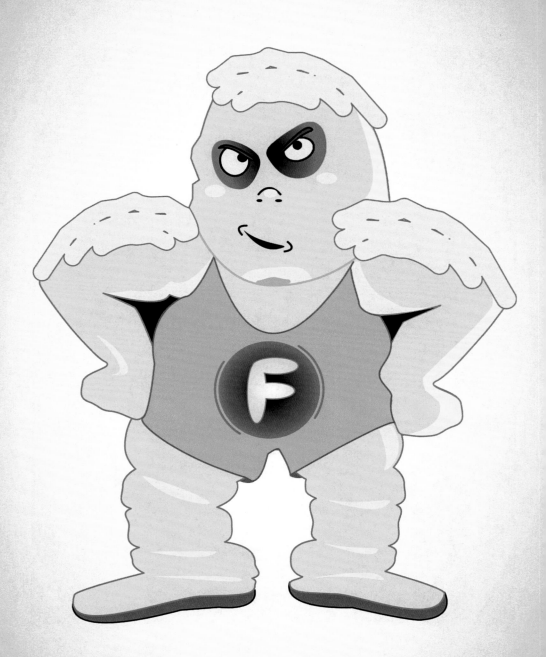

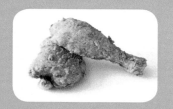 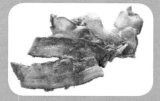 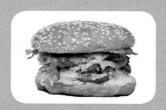

VILLAIN FOOD 4:

Mr. Fat

Where to find him...
✔ Creamy dressing
✔ Fried food
✔ Fast food
✔ Bacon
✔ Cold-cut meats

His Powers...
✔ He will add more fat to your body
✔ He will give you more evil cholesterol
✔ He will weaken your heart
✔ He will zap your energy

QUIZ:
Chapter 3

NAME ————————————

DATE ————————————

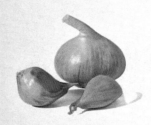

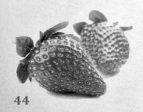

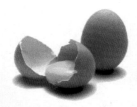

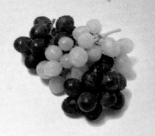

What did you learn?

1. Which **Super Hero(s)** help fight cancer?

_____

2. Which food groups are represented by the **Super Hero Foods**?

_____   _____

_____   _____

3. Give an example of a **SUPER** food:

_____

4. Name 3 things that would be considered **Villain** foods:

_____   _____   _____

5. What is Carotenoid Man's weapon of choice? What does it do?

_____

CHALLENGE:

Using what you have learned, plan a menu for one day. Remember to keep it healthy, simple (doable) and most of all, YUMMY!

(SUPER CHALLENGE – Plan a menu for <u>3</u> days!)

Test your food and nutrition knowledge!

ARE YOU A...

Nutrition
WHIZ KID?

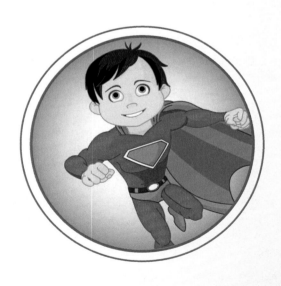

TAKE THE *MATCH IT UP!* **CHALLENGE**

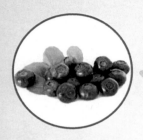

Blueberries

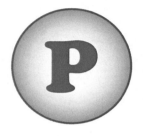

Protein

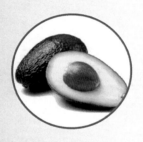

Avocado

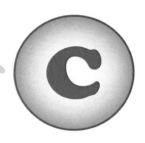

Carbohydrate

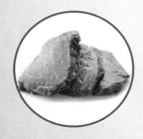

Lean Beef

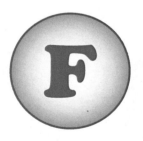

Fat

Match the food with the best nutrient type: Protein, Carbohydrate or Fat.

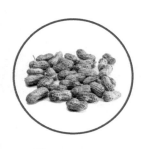

Peanuts

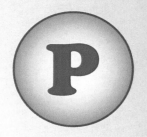

Protein

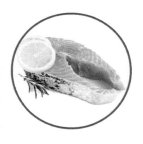

Salmon

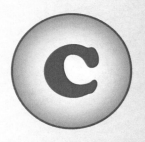

Carbohydrate

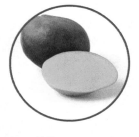

Mango

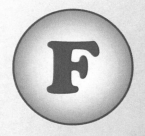

Fat

TAKE THE *MATCH IT UP!* CHALLENGE

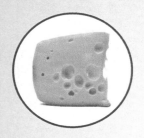

Cheese

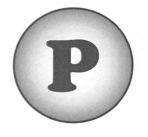

Protein

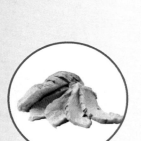

Chicken

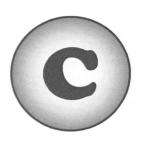

Carbohydrate

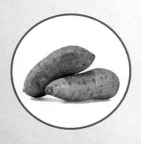

Sweet Potatoes

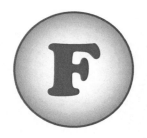

Fat

Match the food with the best nutrient type: Protein, Carbohydrate or Fat.

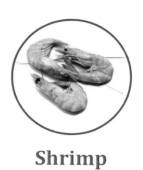

Shrimp

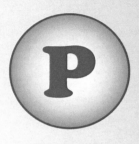

Protein

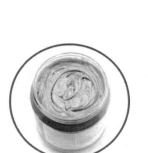

Peanut Butter

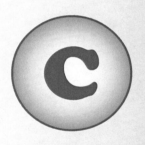

Carbohydrate

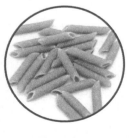

Pasta

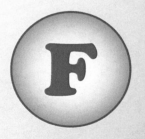

Fat

TAKE THE *MATCH IT UP!*
CHALLENGE

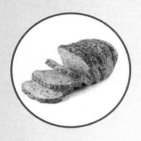

Bread

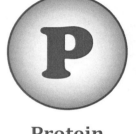

Protein

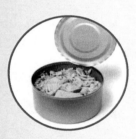

Tuna Fish

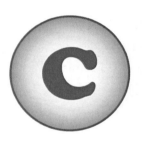

Carbohydrate

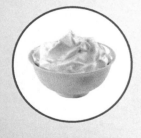

Yogurt

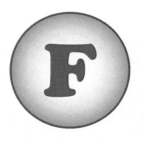

Fat

Match the food with the best nutrient type: Protein, Carbohydrate or Fat.

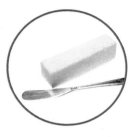

Butter

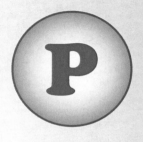

Protein

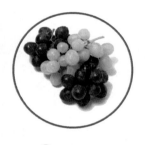

Grapes

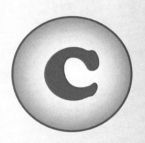

Carbohydrate

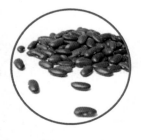

Beans

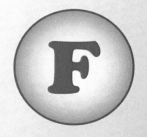

Fat

TAKE THE *MATCH IT UP!*
CHALLENGE

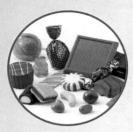

Candy

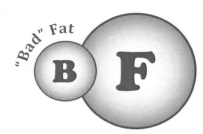

"Bad" Fat

B **F**

Fat

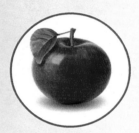

Apple

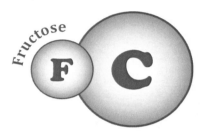

Fructose

F **C**

Carbohydrate

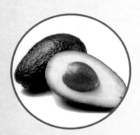

Avocado

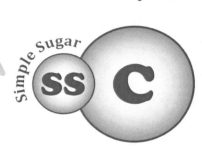

Simple Sugar

SS **C**

Carbohydrate

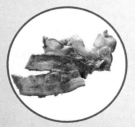

Bacon

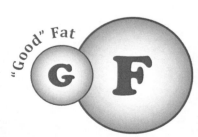

"Good" Fat

G **F**

Fat

Match the food with which the Nutrient type that describes it best.

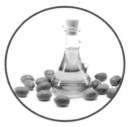

Olive Oil

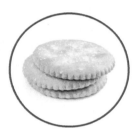

Crackers

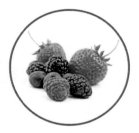

Berries

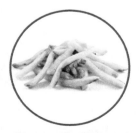

French Fries

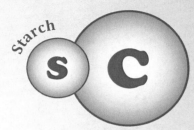

Carbohydrate

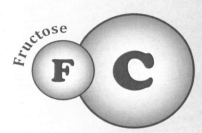

Carbohydrate

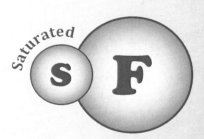

Fat

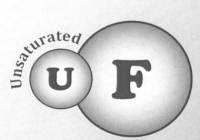

Fat

TAKE THE *MATCH IT UP!* CHALLENGE

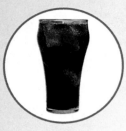

Soda

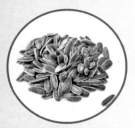

Sunflower Seeds

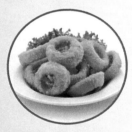

Onion Rings

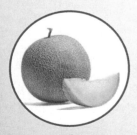

Melon

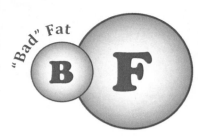

Fat

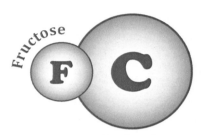

Carbohydrate

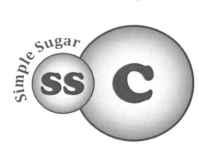

Carbohydrate

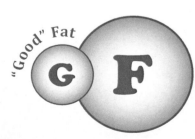

Fat

Match the food with which the Nutrient type that describes it best.

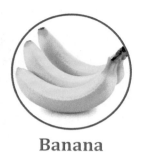

Banana

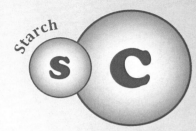

Starch

S **C**

Carbohydrate

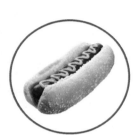

Hot Dog

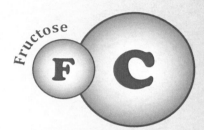

Fructose

F **C**

Carbohydrate

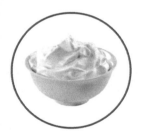

Yogurt

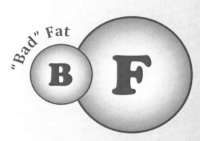

"Bad" Fat

B **F**

Fat

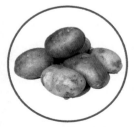

Potatoes

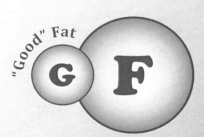

"Good" Fat

G **F**

Fat

TAKE THE *MATCH IT UP!* CHALLENGE

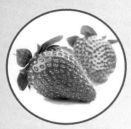

Strawberries

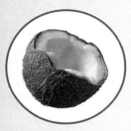

Coconut

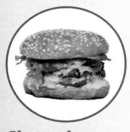

Cheeseburger

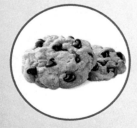

Cookies

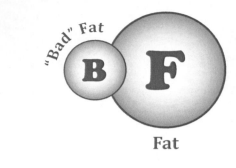

"Bad" Fat

Fat

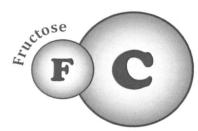

Fructose

Carbohydrate

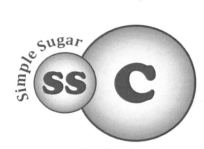

Simple Sugar

Carbohydrate

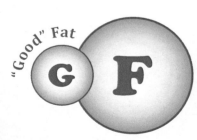

"Good" Fat

Fat

Match the food with which the Nutrient type that describes it best.

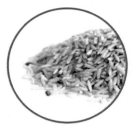

Rice

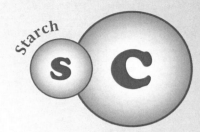

Starch

S **C**

Carbohydrate

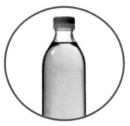

Peanut Oil

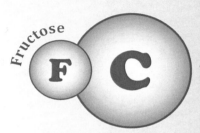

Fructose

F **C**

Carbohydrate

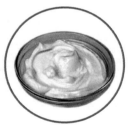

Mayonnaise

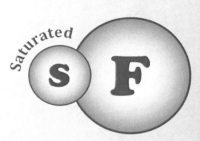

Saturated

S **F**

Fat

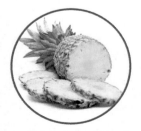

Pineapple

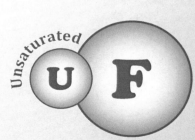

Unsaturated

U **F**

Fat

TAKE THE *MATCH IT UP!* CHALLENGE

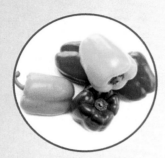

Bell Peppers

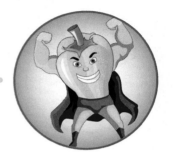

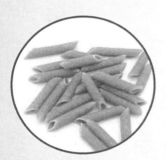

Whole Wheat Pasta

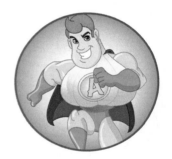

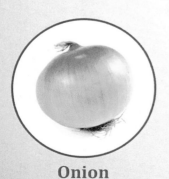

Onion

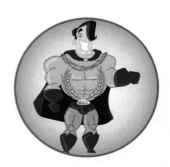

Match the food with the **SUPER HERO (OR VILLAIN).**

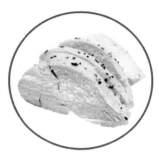

Chicken

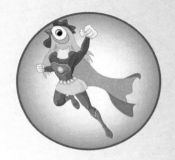

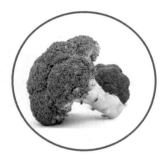

Broccoli

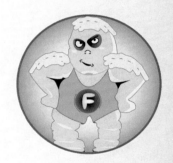

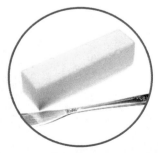

Butter

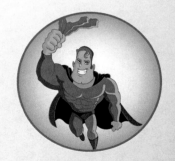

TAKE THE *MATCH IT UP!*
CHALLENGE

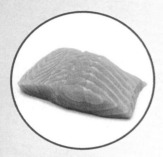

Salmon

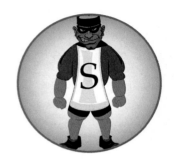

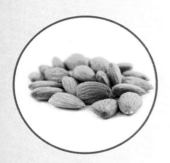

Almonds

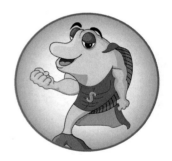

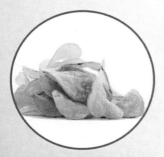

Potato Chips

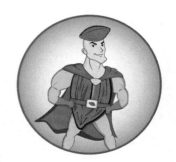

Match the food with the **SUPER HERO (OR VILLAIN).**

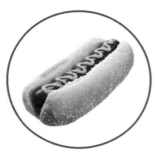

Hot Dog

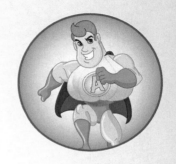

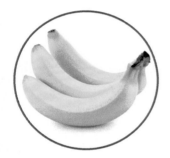

Banana

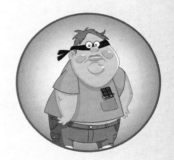

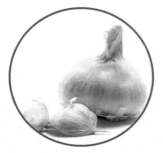

Garlic

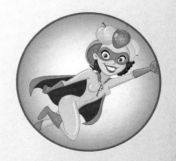

TAKE THE *MATCH IT UP!*
CHALLENGE

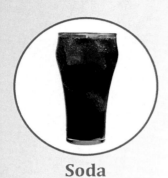

Soda

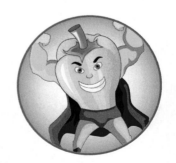

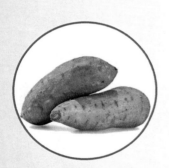

Sweet Potatoes

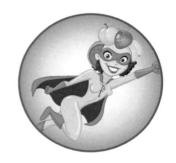

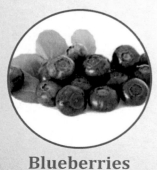

Blueberries

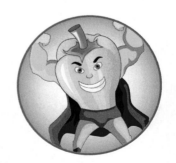

Match the food with the **SUPER HERO (OR VILLAIN).**

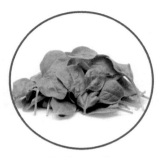

Spinach

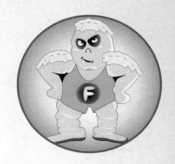

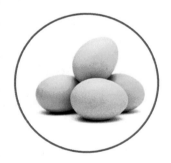

Eggs

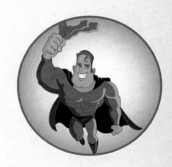

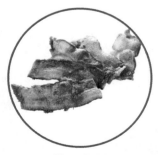

Bacon

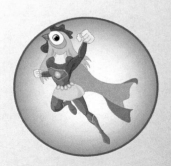

FILL YOUR PLATE!

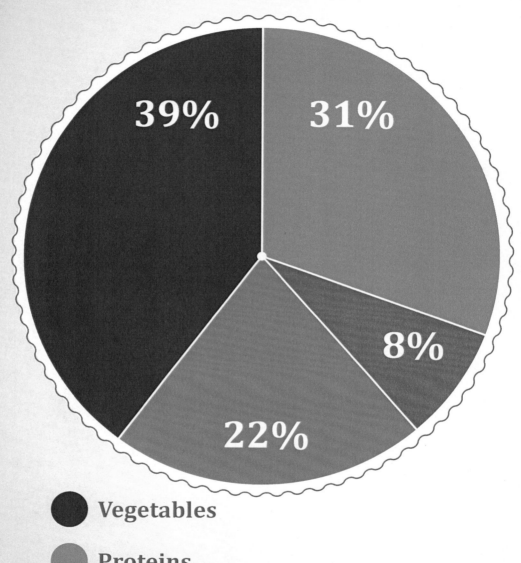

39%   31%   8%   22%

- Vegetables
- Proteins
- Fruits & Grains
- Unsaturated Fats

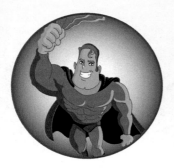 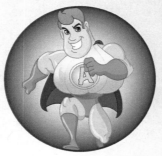 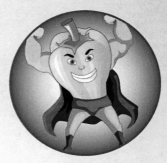

VEGETABLES: The Green Cruciferous Man, Allium Al & Carotenoid Man

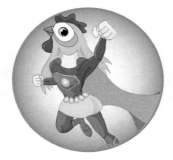 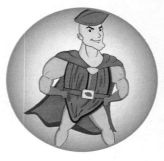 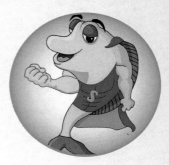

PROTEINS: Poultry Pam, Captain Nut & Seafood Sully

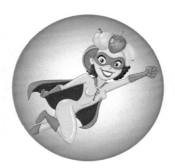 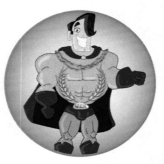

FRUITS & GRAINS: Fruitisha & Whole Grain Harry

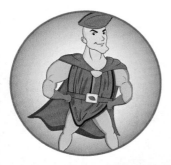

UNSATURATED FATS: Captain Nut

TAKE THE *FILL YOUR PLATE!* CHALLENGE

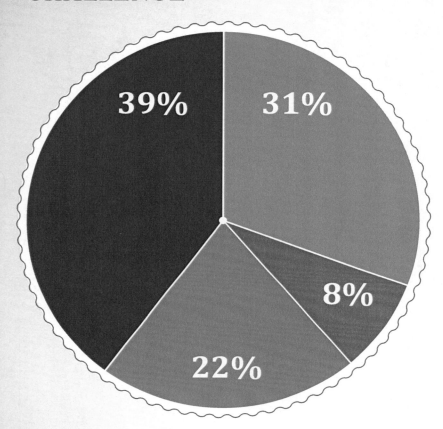

Label the correct plate sections:

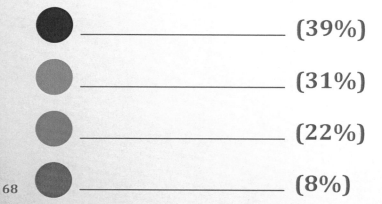

- _____ (39%)
- _____ (31%)
- _____ (22%)
- _____ (8%)

Name at least one **Super Hero Food** for each food group:

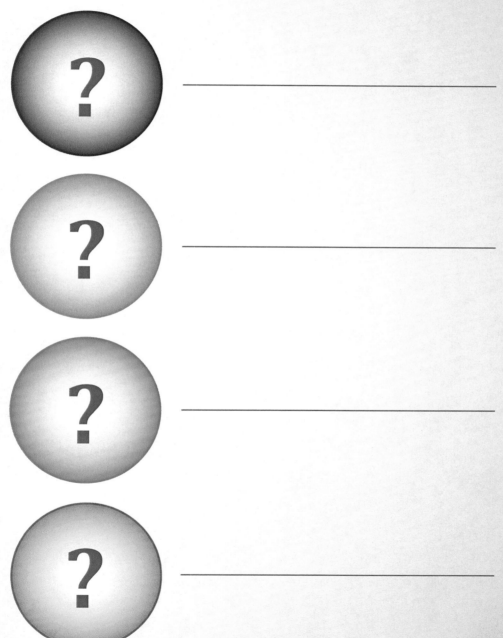

HOW TO READ A NUTRITION LABEL

① **Start here** →

② **Check calories**

③ Limit these nutrients

④ Get enough of these nutrients

⑤ **Footnote**

Sample label for Macaroni & Cheese

Nutrition Facts

Serving Size 1 cup (228g)
Servings Per Container 2

Amount Per Serving

Calories 250   Calories from Fat 110

	% Daily Value*
Total Fat 12g	**18%**
Saturated Fat 3g	**15%**
Trans Fat 3g	
Cholesterol 30mg	**10%**
Sodium 470mg	**20%**
Total Carbohydrate 31g	**10%**
Dietary Fiber 0g	**0%**
Sugars 5g	
Protein 5g	
Vitamin A	**4%**
Vitamin C	**2%**
Calcium	**20%**
Iron	**4%**

* Percent Daily Values are based on a 2,000 calorie diet. Your Daily Values may be higher or lower depending on your calorie needs.

	Calories:	2,000	2,500
Total Fat	Less than	65g	80g
Sat Fat	Less than	20g	25g
Cholesterol	Less than	300mg	300mg
Sodium	Less than	2,400mg	2,400mg
Total Carbohydrate		300g	375g
Dietary Fiber		25g	30g

Quick Guide
to % Daily Value:

• 5% or less is LOW
• 20% or more is HIGH

COOKING HEALTHY, (BUT TASTY) FOR YOUR KIDS

What you eat as a child can affect your eating habits for the duration of your life. During childhood is where most people learn their foundational behaviors that they follow for the remainder of their lives. In other words, if you form poor eating habits as a child there is a relatively good chance that those habits will continue into your teens, and into adulthood. This will most likely pass down from you, to your children, to your children's children.

It is estimated that up to one third of all children in the United States now have a weight problem.* The number of overweight and obese children is growing at an alarming rate and that is simply the fact.

Diseases related to weight gain that were considered adult diseases are now being found in children. Children are now beginning to develop the early signs of clogged arteries, diabetes, and even blood pressure problems. Children who are experiencing high blood pressure at the age of 10 can be expected to have arterial damage by the age of 35.*

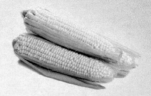

Now is the time to invest in your children and give them the opportunity to develop good eating habits at an early age so they can reduce their chances of obesity. Parents have control over their children's eating habits and food choices. Help your children develop good eating habits give them a gift of good health over a lifetime.

Statistical information was found at:
www.childobesity.com

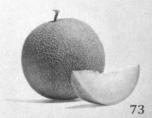

CONVENIENCE OVER NUTRITION

Let's be honest, in the typical household, both parents probably work, and then there is school, homework, soccer, baseball, and church activities. Too often our nutrition is sacrificed due to the convenience of fast food, frozen dinners, and fast casual dining.

It is the responsibility of parents and educators along with culinary professionals to teach children the right nutritional choices and make sure that children are receiving their daily requirement for fresh fruits and vegetables on a daily basis.

If we work together, we can break the chain of bad eating habits and provide children with a foundation of knowledge that will prolong and enrich their lives for years to come!

Check out these resources!

Fruits:
www.choosemyplate.gov/food-groups/fruits_amount_table.html

Vegetables:
www.choosemyplate.gov/food-groups/vegetables_amount_table.html

EAT A RAINBOW EVERY DAY!

Children must learn to *eat a rainbow every day.* Eating a variety of colors is not only interesting to the palate but is important to overall health. Different color fruits and vegetables have different vitamins, minerals, phytonutrients and antioxidants that will help keep your children healthy.

Rather than eating processed foods, we need to encourage fresh, whole foods. Kids need to eat fresh fruits and vegetables and a lot of them! I can hear it now, "Chef Dan, my kids don't eat fruits and vegetables." Yes they will! You may receive some resistance at first but stick with it! You are doing this for them and for their future. As a parent sometimes, you need to present foods in new or fun ways. *Remember, you eat with your eyes first!*

The trick to having children try new foods is to incorporate it into something familiar. For example, most kids love foods like quesadillas, but typically a quesadilla is not the best food choice. What if you made quesadillas with whole wheat tortillas, chicken breast, and added a variety of grilled vegetables? You are then presenting something familiar and introducing something new at the same time.

Another way to introduce nutrition is to hide the vegetables in the food. What kid doesn't love spaghetti and meatballs? Well, a meatball is the perfect way to have your kids eat spinach and enjoy it. That is right, spinach! In your regular meatball mix, add a pack of frozen spinach, which has been drained and squeezed of the water. If you are purchasing frozen meatballs, try making them! You will save a lot of money, and you will know exactly what is in what you are feeding your family.

FOOD SHOULD BE FUN!

The easiest way to have a child try new foods is to have them get involved! From an early age, I was drawn to cook by my mother, an amazing cook who was always able to create something from nothing by turning the most basic ingredients into an amazing meal. She noticed my interest in food as a young child and began to show me how to make easy recipes. She taught me to make healthy, home cooked meals with what was available and instilled in me a passion for cooking that quickly grew.

So many times I hear a parent say to their child "You don't like that." If you take anything away from this section then, as a parent, remove that from your vocabulary. Always encourage your children to try new things and introduce them to new opportunities every chance you get! Life is about new experiences and you are doing this for them and for their future. Food is so much more than just what we eat. It is our culture, our company, our comfort, and our inspiration.

"It is very challenging at times to ensure that my children are eating healthy, well-balanced meals. They are drawn towards the highly palatable, high fat, highly preservative-containing foods, and as a working parent I am drawn towards the same for their convenience. It is imperative though, to teach them at a young age how to make healthy choices, so that they will carry that knowledge with them into adulthood and enjoy a healthy lifestyle. The challenge is to make the transition, change the faulty choices, and set them on the correct path. Even at a very young age, children have the capacity to understand food groups and making healthy choices. We will often make a game at dinner, seeing if food from each of the four groups is on their plate....and if it is not, we try a way to incorporate the missing group. There will undoubtedly be resistance, as there was in our home. But persistence will pay off, as it was not too long before the children not only accepted the new norm, but found the healthy foods to be highly palatable. And that is a great gift to have given them."
–Samara Friedman, Short Hills, NJ (food by dan client).

Chef Dan Vogt is the owner of "food by dan" and "Eat to Lose Foods." Chef Dan's services operate on a national level. For more information about Chef Dan and his services please visit **foodbydan.com** and/or **eattolosefoods.com.**

Below are a few fun and tasty recipes that you and your children can make together! I hope this helps encourage healthy eating habits in you and your children's lives! **Remember, food should be fun and a recipe's potential only stops at your imagination!**

BLACKBERRY GINGER BREAKFAST SMOOTHIE

Ingredients:

- 2 cups of ice
- 24 oz. of water
- 2 cups of unsweetened blackberries
- 1/2 cup plain non-fat yogurt
- 1 tsp. fresh grated ginger
- 4 TB of honey
- 1 scoop of French vanilla whey protein (optional)

Place all of the ingredients in a blender and blend for five minutes. Serve in glasses with a straw.

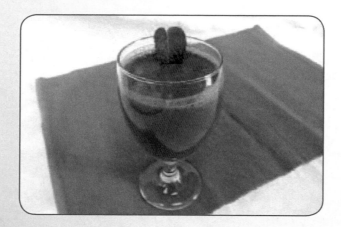

Calories (kcal):..257
% of Calories from Fat: 2.5%
% of Calories from Carbohydrates:....................................86.7%
% of Calories from Protein: 10.8%

Per Serving Nutritional Information

Total Fat (g):	1 g	1%	Vitamin B12 (mcg):	1.0mcg	17%
Saturated Fat (g):	trace	1%	Thiamin B1 (mg):	.2 mg	15%
Monounsaturated Fat (g):	trace	1%	Riboflavin B2 (mg):	.9 mg	53%
Polyunsaturated Fat (g):	trace	1%	Folacin (mcg):	34 mcg	8%
Cholesterol Fat (mg):	3mg	1%	Niacin (mg):	1 mg	7%
Total Carbohydrate (g):	59 g	20%	Caffeine (mg):	0 mg	N/A
Dietary Fiber (g):	4 g	15%	Alcohol (kcal):	0	N/A
Protein (g):	7 g	15%			
Sodium (mg):	423 mg	18%	**Food Exchanges**		
Potassium (mg):	945 mg	27%	Grain (Starch):		0
Calcium (mg):	374 mg	37%	Lean Meat:		1/2
Iron (mg):	1 mg	6%	Vegetable:		0
Zinc (mg):	1 mg	8%	Fruit:		1
Vitamin C (mg):	3 mg	5%	Non-Fat Milk:		0
Vitamin A (i.u.):	104 IU	2%	Fat:		0
Vitamin A (r.e.):	23 RE	1%	Other Carbohydrates:		3
Vitamin B6 (mg):	.3 mg	14%			

* Percent Daily Values are based on a 2000 calorie diet

Nutrition Facts

Serving Size 7 1/10 oz (202.0 g)

Amount Per Serving

Calories 560   Calories from Fat 288

	% Daily Value*
Total Fat 32.0g	**49%**
Saturated Fat 12.0g	**60%**
Cholesterol 265mg	**88%**
Sodium 1360mg	**57%**
Total Carbohydrates 48.0g	**16%**
Dietary Fiber 2.0g	**8%**
Sugars 15.0g	
Protein 20.0g	

Vitamin A 10%	•	Vitamin C 0%
Calcium 20%	•	Iron 15%

* Based on a 2000 calorie diet

◀ **Compare to a typical fast food pancake, sausage, and egg sandwich.**

TURKEY BURGERS WITH LETTUCE BUNS

Ingredients

- 1 lb. lean ground turkey
- 1 tsp. of your favorite BBQ seasoning (no sugar)
- 2 tsp. low-sodium worcestershire sauce
- 2 tsp. low-sodium soy sauce
- 16 red romaine lettuce leaves (darker the better)

Suggested toppings (have fun!)

- red onion
- tomatoes
- dill pickle chips
- avocado

Mix turkey and seasonings together. Form into 4-ounce patties. Grill, sauté, or bake burgers until they have the internal temperature of 165 degrees. Serve burgers with lettuce leaves as buns and a variety of toppings.

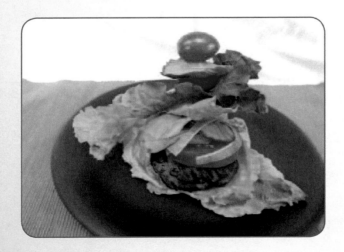

Calories (kcal):			301

Calories (kcal):...301
% of Calories from Fat: 35.8%
% of Calories from Carbohydrates:...29.6%
% of Calories from Protein: 34.6%

Per Serving Nutritional Information

Total Fat (g):	13 g	20%		Vitamin B12 (mcg):	0mcg	0%
Saturated Fat (g):	3 g	14%		Thiamin B1 (mg):	.2 mg	13%
Monounsaturated Fat (g):	3 g	11%		Riboflavin B2 (mg):	.2 mg	9%
Polyunsaturated Fat (g):	1 g	4%		Folacin (mcg):	119 mcg	30%
Cholesterol Fat (mg):	73mg	24%		Niacin (mg):	2 mg	9%
Total Carbohydrate (g):	24 g	8%		Caffeine (mg):	0 mg	N/A
Dietary Fiber (g):	6 g	23%		Alcohol (kcal):	0	N/A
Protein (g):	28 g	55%				
Sodium (mg):	409 mg	17%		**Food Exchanges**		
Potassium (mg):	812 mg	23%		Grain (Starch):		0
Calcium (mg):	57 mg	6%		Lean Meat:		3 1/2
Iron (mg):	2 mg	10%		Vegetable:		4
Zinc (mg):	1 mg	4%		Fruit:		0
Vitamin C (mg):	46 mg	76%		Non-Fat Milk:		0
Vitamin A (i.u.):	2249 IU	45%		Fat:		1
Vitamin A (r.e.):	224.5 RE	22%		Other Carbohydrates:		0
Vitamin B6 (mg):	.3 mg	17%				

* Percent Daily Values are based on a 2000 calorie diet

Nutrition Facts

Serving Size 1 Serving (190.0 g)

Amount Per Serving

Calories 550	Calories from Fat 288
	% Daily Value*
Total Fat 32.0g	**49%**
Saturated Fat 15.0g	**75%**
Cholesterol 85mg	**28%**
Sodium 690mg	**29%**
Total Carbohydrates 39.5g	**13%**
Dietary Fiber 2.0g	**8%**
Sugars 8.5g	
Protein 27.0g	

* Based on a 2000 calorie diet

◄ Compare to a typical casual dine-in burger

PEPPERONI PIZZA KABOBS

Ingredients:

- 4 slices of turkey pepperoni
- 8 small fresh mozzarella (1" diameter)
- 16 chunks of bell pepper
- 12 cherry or grape tomatoes
- 4 basil leaves
- 4 wood skewers

Cut bell peppers into 1" x 1" chunks. Slice pepperoni in half. Slice basil leaves in half. Assemble ingredients onto skewers and enjoy!

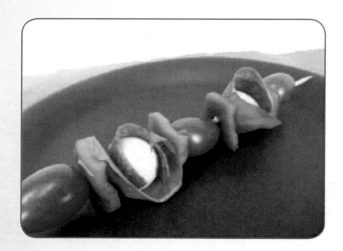

Calories (kcal):.. 78
% of Calories from Fat: 43.6%
% of Calories from Carbohydrates:...22.2%
% of Calories from Protein: 34.2%

Per Serving Nutritional Information

Total Fat (g):	4 g	6%	Vitamin B12 (mcg):	.2mcg	3%
Saturated Fat (g):	2 g	11%	Thiamin B1 (mg):	trace	3%
Monounsaturated Fat (g):	1 g	5%	Riboflavin B2 (mg):	.1 mg	4%
Polyunsaturated Fat (g):	trace	1%	Folacin (mcg):	15 mcg	4%
Cholesterol Fat (mg):	15 mg	5%	Niacin (mg):	trace	2%
Total Carbohydrate (g):	4 g	1%	Caffeine (mg):	0 mg	N/A
Dietary Fiber (g):	1 g	4%	Alcohol (kcal):	0	N/A
Protein (g):	7 g	14%			
Sodium (mg):	179 mg	7%	**Food Exchanges**		
Potassium (mg):	174 mg	5%	Grain (Starch):		0
Calcium (mg):	142 mg	14%	Lean Meat:		1/2
Iron (mg):	trace	2%	Vegetable:		1/2
Zinc (mg):	1 mg	4%	Fruit:		0
Vitamin C (mg):	31 mg	51%	Non-Fat Milk:		0
Vitamin A (i.u.):	601 IU	12%	Fat:		0
Vitamin A (r.e.):	84 RE	8%	Other Carbohydrates:		0
Vitamin B6 (mg):	.1 mg	5%			

* Percent Daily Values are based on a 2000 calorie diet

Nutrition Facts

Serving Size 6 rolls (0.1 g)

Amount Per Serving

Calories 210	Calories from Fat 90
	% Daily Value*
Total Fat 10.0g	**15%**
Saturated Fat 3.0g	**15%**
Trans Fat 1.5g	
Cholesterol 10mg	**3%**
Sodium 450mg	**19%**
Total Carbohydrates 24.0g	**8%**
Dietary Fiber 1.0g	**4%**
Sugars 2.0g	
Protein 7.0g	
Vitamin A 6%	Vitamin C 0%
Calcium 2%	Iron 8%

* Based on a 2000 calorie diet

◀ Compare to frozen mini pizza rolls

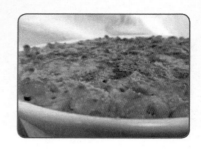

HEALTHY MACARONI AND CHEESE

Ingredients (8 servings):

- 1 lb. whole wheat elbow pasta
- 1 head cauliflower
- 2 cups 1% low fat milk
- 6 oz. extra sharp cheddar cheese
- 1/2 cup part skim ricotta cheese
- 1 tsp. Kosher salt
- 1/2 tsp. black pepper
- 1/8 tsp. nutmeg
- 1 TB dijon mustard
- 1/8 tsp. cayenne pepper
- 2 TB grated parmesan cheese
- 1 tsp. extra virgin olive oil
- 1 minced onion
- 3 cloves minced garlic

1. Bring a pot of salted water to a boil. Place chopped cauliflower into the boiling pot of water until fork tender.

2. In a separate pan, sauté the onions, garlic, and spices with olive oil. Once the onions are translucent, add dijon mustard and milk. Bring to a simmer.

3. Add cheddar and ricotta cheese, whisk until incorporated.

4. Drain cauliflower, add pasta to boiling water.

5. Blend sauce and cooked cauliflower with stick blender or in a food processor.

6. Drain pasta; mix with sauce in a baking dish, top with parmesan cheese.

7. Bake at 425 for 20 minutes or until the crust is golden brown.

Calories (kcal):	313
% of Calories from Fat:	26.5%
% of Calories from Carbohydrates:	53.4%
% of Calories from Protein:	20.1%

Per Serving Nutritional Information

Total Fat (g):	10 g	15%	Vitamin B12 (mcg):	.4mcg	7%
Saturated Fat (g):	5 g	27%	Thiamin B1 (mg):	.3 mg	19%
Monounsaturated Fat (g):	3 g	15%	Riboflavin B2 (mg):	.3 mg	16%
Polyunsaturated Fat (g):	1 g	3%	Folacin (mcg):	46 mcg	11%
Cholesterol Fat (mg):	27 mg	9%	Niacin (mg):	3 mg	14%
Total Carbohydrate (g):	44 g	15%	Caffeine (mg):	0 mg	N/A
Dietary Fiber (g):	5 g	19%	Alcohol (kcal):	0	N/A
Protein (g):	16 g	33%			
Sodium (mg):	420 mg	18%	**Food Exchanges**		
Potassium (mg):	291 mg	8%	Grain (Starch):		2 1/2
Calcium (mg):	284 mg	28%	Lean Meat:		1
Iron (mg):	2 mg	12%	Vegetable:		1/2
Zinc (mg):	2 mg	15%	Fruit:		0
Vitamin C (mg):	7 mg	11%	Non-Fat Milk:		0
Vitamin A (i.u.):	391 IU	8%	Fat:		1 1/2
Vitamin A (r.e.):	114.5 RE	11%	Other Carbohydrates:		0
Vitamin B6 (mg):	.2 mg	10%			

Percent Daily Values are based on a 2000 calorie diet

Nutrition Facts

Serving Size 1 serving (g)

Amount Per Serving

Calories 510   Calories from Fat 162

% Daily Value*

Total Fat 18.0g	**28%**
Saturated Fat 6.0g	**30%**
Sodium 940mg	**39%**
Total Carbohydrates 69.0g	**23%**
Dietary Fiber 3.0g	**12%**
Protein 16.0g	

* Based on a 2000 calorie diet

◀ Compare to Macaroni and Cheese Kid's Meal (excluding side) from national chain bar and grill

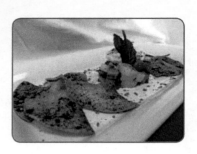

DESSERT NACHOS

Ingredients (2 servings):

Chips:
- 4 soft corn tortillas
- 1/4 tsp. cinnamon
- 1/8 tsp. stevia sweetener (Truvia)
- olive oil spray
- 4 wood skewers

Salsa:
- 1/2 cup chopped berries (tomatoes)
- 1/2 cup chopped kiwi (peppers)
- 1/2 cup chopped jicama (onions)
- 1 tsp. lime juice
- 1 tsp. chopped mint (cilantro)
- 1/2 tsp. honey

Toppings:
- 2 tsp. non-fat, plain yogurt (sour cream)
- 1 tsp. 70% cocoa dark chocolate (shredded cheese)

1. Cut tortillas in to 4 even triangles and scatter on a sheet pan.

2. Spray tortillas with olive oil spray.

3. Sprinkle with cinnamon and stevia sweetener, then bake at 350 until crispy (usually 20 minutes).

4. Chop and mix ingredients for salsa (fruit, mint, honey, lime juice).

5. Top chips with salsa, yogurt, and dark chocolate shavings.

Calories (kcal):	....	182
% of Calories from Fat:	....	11.6%
% of Calories from Carbohydrates:	....	79.7%
% of Calories from Protein:	....	8.7%

Per Serving Nutritional Information

Total Fat (g):	3 g	4%	Vitamin B12 (mcg):	trace	0%
Saturated Fat (g):	trace	1%	Thiamin B1 (mg):	.1 mg	4%
Monounsaturated Fat (g):	trace	2%	Riboflavin B2 (mg):	.1 mg	4%
Polyunsaturated Fat (g):	1 g	3%	Folacin (mcg):	66 mcg	16%
Cholesterol Fat (mg):	trace	0%	Niacin (mg):	1 mg	6%
Total Carbohydrate (g):	39 g	13%	Caffeine (mg):	1 mg	N/A
Dietary Fiber (g):	7 g	27%	Alcohol (kcal):	0	N/A
Protein (g):	4 g	9%			
Sodium (mg):	89 mg	4%	**Food Exchanges**		
Potassium (mg):	358 mg	10%	Grain (Starch):		1 1/2
Calcium (mg):	123 mg	12%	Lean Meat:		0
Iron (mg):	1 mg	8%	Vegetable:		0
Zinc (mg):	1 mg	5%	Fruit:		1/2
Vitamin C (mg):	66 mg	109%	Non-Fat Milk:		0
Vitamin A (i.u.):	134 IU	3%	Fat:		1/2
Vitamin A (r.e.):	13.5 RE	1%	Other Carbohydrates:		0
Vitamin B6 (mg):	.1 mg	6%			

* Percent Daily Values are based on a 2000 calorie diet

Nutrition Facts

Serving Size 1 sundae (203.0 g)

Amount Per Serving

Calories 530   Calories from Fat 261

           % Daily Value*

Total Fat 29.0g	**45%**
Saturated Fat 19.0g	**95%**
Cholesterol 85mg	**28%**
Sodium 200mg	**8%**
Total Carbohydrates 62.0g	**21%**
Sugars 52.0g	
Protein 8.0g	

Vitamin A 15%	•	Vitamin C 2%
Calcium 20%	•	Iron 2%

* Based on a 2000 calorie diet

◄ Compare to
Hot Fudge Sundae
from national
ice cream chain

ENERGY MUFFINS

Finally, a great-tasting muffin recipe with no added sugar! Naturally sweetened with banana and blueberries, these muffins are as sweet as they are delicious. Enjoy one with a side of scrambled egg whites for a quick and nutritious breakfast. **Servings: 18**

Ingredients:

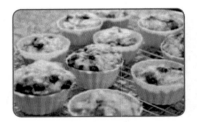

- 1 cup mashed banana
- 2 egg whites
- 1/2 cup water
- 1/3 cup refined coconut oil
- 2 cups wheat flour
- 1 tsp. baking soda
- 2 $1/4$ tsp. baking powder
- 1 cup frozen blueberries, left to thaw in a strainer

1. Preheat oven to 350 degrees. Prepare 18 standard sized muffin cups with paper liners.

2. In a large bowl, combine banana, egg whites, water and oil. Add the flour and mix. Gently fold in blueberries. Immediately spoon batter into muffin cups.

3. Bake for about 20 minutes. Remove muffins from tins and cool on a wire rack.

Nutritional Analysis:
One serving equals: 98 calories, 4g fat, 13g carbohydrate, 2g fiber, and 3g protein.

FASTEST CHICKEN STIR FRY

Think you don't have enough time to cook a healthy meal? Think again. This healthy and delicious chicken stir fry takes only minutes to make. Instead of chopping the vegetables yourself, this recipe calls for pre-chopped ingredients found in the produce section of your grocery store. Skip the take-out line tonight and try this recipe instead. **Servings: 6**

Ingredients:

- 1 tsp. olive oil
- 1 tsp. chopped garlic
- 1 cup asparagus, cut into 2 inch segments
- 1 (16 oz.) package pre-chopped stir fry vegetables
- 1 (10 oz.) package shredded cabbage
- 1 cup chopped pineapple
- 1 cup chopped cooked chicken breast
- 3/4 cup teriyaki sauce

1. Heat the olive oil in a large skillet or wok. Add the garlic. When the garlic is browned add the asparagus. Stir fry for 5 minutes or until the asparagus turns bright green.

2. Add the chopped stir fry vegetables, cabbage, and pineapple. Stir fry for 5 minutes or until the vegetables are tender.

3. Add the cooked chicken pieces and mix in the teriyaki sauce. Stir fry for another minute, until the sauce is evenly distributed.

Nutritional Analysis:
One serving equals: 117 calories, 1.8g fat, 15.8g carbohydrate, 4g fiber, and 10.7g protein.

QUICK CHICKEN AND VEGGIE BOWL

This recipe serves up a refreshing new twist on chicken. Delicious veggies and chunks of tender chicken are coated in a savory sauce, and served over wild rice. It works great as a weekday meal, since it only takes about 20 minutes to make.
Servings: 6

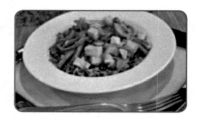

Ingredients:

- 2 cups wild rice, cooked
- 1 TB sesame oil
- 1 sweet potato, halved and thinly sliced
- 1/2 cup red onion, thinly sliced
- 1 cup mushroom, sliced
- 1 TB ginger root, minced
- 3 cloves garlic, minced
- 2 TB mirin (rice cooking wine)
- 2 TB soy sauce
- 1 TB toasted sesame oil
- 1 tsp. corn starch
- 1/2 tsp. rushed red pepper
- 2 cups green beans, chopped
- 4 cups chicken breast, cooked and cubed

1. In a large saucepan place the sesame oil over medium heat. Add the sweet potato, onion, mushroom, ginger and garlic. Sauté for 5 minutes.

2. In a small bowl combine the mirin, soy sauce, toasted sesame oil, cornstarch and red pepper. Set aside.

3. Add the green beans and chicken into the pan and continue to cook for 2 minutes. Pour the soy sauce mixture in and mix until fully incorporated. Cook for another 3 minutes.

4. Serve over wild rice.

Nutritional Analysis:
One serving equals: 299 calories, 8g fat, 23g carbohydrate, 2g fiber, and 33g protein.

GUILTLESS ZUCCHINI PASTA WITH TURKEY

Here is a guiltless way to prepare spaghetti that the whole family will love. To create angel hair noodles out of zucchini you simply need a small kitchen gadget called a spiral slicer. This ingenious tool is well worth the small investment— with it you'll quickly and easily make delicious, fiber-filled noodles. **Servings: 4**

Ingredients:

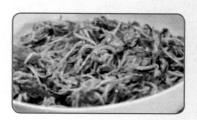

- 4 zucchini, ends trimmed and run through a spiral slicer
- 1 tsp. olive oil
- 1/2 cup chopped onion
- 3 garlic cloves, minced
- 1 (20 oz.) package lean ground turkey
- 2 cups spaghetti sauce
- salt and pepper to taste

1. Place the spiral-sliced zucchini in a large bowl and set aside.

2. In a medium sized skillet heat the oil. Add the onion and garlic and sauté until soft.

3. Add the turkey to the skillet and cook until fully browned. Add the spaghetti sauce and mix until fully incorporated. Remove from heat.

4. Mix the sauce with the zucchini noodles in the large bowl and serve.

Nutritional Analysis:
One serving equals: 292 calories, 8g fat, 26g carbohydrate, 5g fiber, and 27g protein.

FIRE-ROASTED CHILE OMELET

Here's a recipe to spice up your breakfast. Egg whites, fire-roasted green chile and diced tomatoes create a tasty omelet that is bursting with flavor and packed with protein. Serve with a side of salsa and sliced avocado. **Servings: 2**

Ingredients:

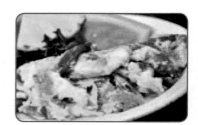

- 1 tsp. olive oil
- 3 small tomatoes, finely chopped
- 2 (4 oz.) cans of fire-roasted, diced green chiles
- 12 egg whites
- 2 TB water
- non-stick cooking spray

1. In a skillet, heat the oil over medium heat. Add the tomatoes and chiles and cook until soft, about 3 minutes. Season with pepper and salt and set aside.

2. In a medium bowl whisk the egg whites and water. Lightly coat a medium non-stick skillet with non-stick cooking spray and place over medium heat. Add 1/4 of the eggs and swirl to evenly coat the bottom of that pan. Cook until the eggs have set, about 2 minutes.

3. Use a rubber scraper to lift the eggs up and let the runny uncooked egg flow underneath. Spoon 1/4 of the Chile mixture onto half of the omelet, fold over, and slide onto a serving plate. Repeat with remaining egg whites and Chile mixture.

Nutritional Analysis:
One serving equals: 163 calories, 5g fat, 6g carbohydrate, 2g fiber, and 26g protein.

HERB-COATED HALIBUT WITH ZUCCHINI AND WHOLE WHEAT COUSCOUS

Not only is this meal delicious, it's also incredibly healthy. A tangy herb paste coats both the fish and zucchini, which roast on the same pan. The entire meal is ready in 30 minutes—perfect for busy weekday dinners. **Servings: 4**

Ingredients:

- 6 scallions, chopped
- 1 cup packed fresh cilantro
- 1/2 cup packed fresh mint
- 3 TB olive oil
- 1 TB chopped, peeled fresh ginger
- 3/4 tsp. ground coriander
- salt and pepper to taste
- 1 zucchini, cut into spears
- 4 skinless fillets firm white fish
- 1 cup dry whole-wheat couscous

1. Preheat oven to 425 degrees. Throw the scallions, cilantro, mint, oil, ginger, coriander and 1/2 teaspoon salt into a food processor and pulse until a coarse paste forms. Season with pepper.

2. Toss zucchini with 3 tablespoons herb paste in a bowl. Spread onto a rimmed baking sheet. Roast for 5 minutes.

3. Rub remaining herb paste onto both sides of fish fillets. Push zucchini to edges of baking sheet, and arrange fish in center, leaving about 1/2 inch between each fillet. Roast until fish is opaque and semi-firm to the touch, about 15 minutes. Meanwhile, prepare couscous according to directions.

4. Serve fish and zucchini over couscous.

Nutritional Analysis:
One serving equals: 354 calories, 10g fat, 29g carbohydrate, 6g fiber, and 32g protein.

CHICKEN QUINOA STIR FRY

Here is a simple, wholesome meal that is ready in 30 minutes—perfect for busy weekday dinners. There's no reason to hit the take-out line when you have this quick and delicious recipe on hand. **Servings: 4**

Ingredients:

- 1 cup cooked quinoa
- 1 tsp. olive oil
- 1/2 onion, chopped
- 1 clove garlic, minced
- 1/2 red bell pepper, chopped
- 1/2 green bell pepper, chopped
- 1/2 yellow bell pepper, chopped
- 1 ear of corn, kernels cut from cob
- handful of asparagus stalks, cut into 1 inch pieces
- 2 cups baked chicken breast, cut into small cubes
- 1 can of organic black beans, drained and rinsed
- splash of lemon juice
- splash of lime juice
- dash of salt and pepper
- splash of soy sauce
- 1/4 cup fresh parsley, finely chopped

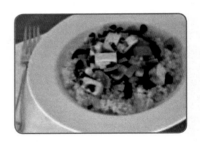

1. Cook the quinoa and set aside. Place a large saucepan over medium heat. Add the oil, onion and garlic. Sauté for about 3 minutes. Add the bell peppers, corn and asparagus, cook until the vegetables are tender. Add the chicken and beans, cook for another 10 minutes, adding the rest of the ingredients.

2. Place a serving of quinoa on each plate and top it with the vegetable mix.

Nutritional Analysis:
One serving equals: 293 calories, 5g fat, 32g carbohydrate, 4.6g fiber, and 29.4g protein.

SPINACH AND EGG WHITE WRAP

This wrap is delicious for breakfast, lunch or dinner. It's ready in a flash, tastes amazing, and is filled with lean protein, veggies and whole sprouted grains. Try it today, but don't be surprised if you get hooked! **Servings: 2**

Ingredients:

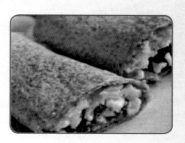

- 1 tsp. olive oil
- 1 garlic clove, minced
- 3/4 cup tomato, finely chopped
- 2 cups spinach, roughly chopped
- 1 cup egg whites
- dash of salt and pepper
- 2 sprouted grain tortillas
- 2 TB pesto *(Purchase it pre-made, or combine 1/2 cup walnuts, 2 cups basil leaves, 2 cloves garlic, 1/4 cup olive oil, and 1 TB lemon juice in a food processor and blend until it becomes a paste.)*

1. Spread 1 TB of pesto over each tortilla and set aside.

2. In medium sized skillet warm the olive oil over medium heat. Add the garlic and sauté until golden. Add the tomato and cook for another 3 minutes. Add the spinach and cook until it is soft and wilted. Remove the veggies from skillet, set aside in a bowl.

3. Pour the egg whites into the skillet, season with salt and pepper. Cook until the egg is no longer runny.

4. Arrange half of the egg whites in a line down the center of each tortilla. Top with half of the veggies and then fold the ends up and wrap like a burrito.

Nutritional Analysis:
One serving equals: 288 calories, 10g fat, 28g carbohydrate, 6g fiber, and 21g protein.

EASY TERIYAKI SALMON

Salmon is filled with healthy omega 3 essential fatty acids, protein, and vitamin B12. This recipe is quick and tastes amazing. Serve it with a side of brown rice and steamed veggies. **Servings: 4**

Ingredients:

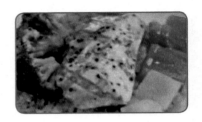

1 TB sesame oil
1/4 cup lemon juice
1/4 cup soy sauce
1 tsp. ground mustard
1 tsp. ground ginger
1/4 tsp. garlic powder
4 (6 oz.) salmon steaks

1. In a large re-sealable plastic bag combine the first six ingredients; mix well.

2. Set aside 1/2 cup of marinade and refrigerate.

3. Add salmon to remaining marinade, cover and refrigerate for 1-1/2 hours, turning once. Drain and discard marinade.

4. Place the salmon on a broiler pan. Broil 3-4 in. from the heat for 5 minutes. Brush with reserved marinade; turn and broil for 5 minutes or until fish flakes easily with a fork. Brush with remaining marinade.

Nutritional Analysis:
One serving equals: 392 calories, 19g fat, 2.6g carbohydrate, .2g fiber, and 38g protein.

HEALTHY CHOCOLATE SHAKE

What is better than a creamy chocolate shake? A creamy chocolate shake without the guilt! You won't miss the fat and refined sugar as you slurp up this tasty treat. **Servings: 2**

Ingredients:

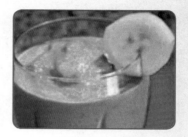

- 2 bananas, frozen
- 1 packet of plain instant oatmeal
- 1/2 cup nonfat milk
- 2 scoops chocolate whey protein
- 2 TB raw almond butter
- dash of ground cinnamon
- 2 cups ice

1. Put all ingredients into a high speed blender. Blend until smooth and creamy.

Nutritional Analysis:

One serving equals: 292 calories, 7g fat, 33g carbohydrate, 7g fiber, and 25g protein.

BONUS BREAKFAST RECIPE!

HEALTHY PROTEIN-POWERED PANCAKES FOR KIDS

Ingredients:

- 1 cup of egg whites
- 1 whole egg
- 1/2 cup of oatmeal
- 1 cup of blueberries
- sprinkle of cinnamon
- 2 packets of Stevia (optional)

Whip in a blender and pour on the griddle to make pancakes. You can serve with agave nectar.

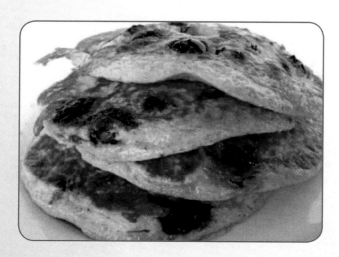

Get Creative!

▶ Use this page to record your own
  HEALTHY BUT TASTY recipe ideas!

_____

_____

_____

_____

_____

_____

_____

_____

_____

_____

_____